This Fitness Journal Belongs to:

	Calories	Carbs	Fat	Protein
Breakfast:				
Lunch:				
Dinner:				
Snack:				
Daily Total:				

Water Intake

To Do:

☐
☐
☐
☐
☐

Daily Goals:

____

____

____

____

Date:

Work Out

Exercise	Duration	Intensity

Current Weight _______________

Met Goals Today?   Yes   No
                      O   O

Notes

____

____

____

____

____

____

____

____

____

	Calories	Carbs	Fat	Protein
Breakfast:				
Lunch:				
Dinner:				
Snack:				
Daily Total:				

Water Intake

To Do:

- ☐
- ☐
- ☐
- ☐
- ☐

Daily Goals:

Date:

Work Out

Exercise	Duration	Intensity

Current Weight ___________________

Met Goals Today?   Yes   No
                      O   O

Notes

____

____

____

____

____

____

____

____

____

____

	Calories	Carbs	Fat	Protein
Breakfast:				
Lunch:				
Dinner:				
Snack:				
Daily Total:				

Water Intake

To Do:

☐
☐
☐
☐
☐

Daily Goals:

____

____

____

____

Date:

Work Out

Exercise	Duration	Intensity

Current Weight _______________

Met Goals Today?   Yes O   No O

Notes

____

____

____

____

____

____

____

____

____

	Calories	Carbs	Fat	Protein
Breakfast:				
Lunch:				
Dinner:				
Snack:				
Daily Total:				

Water Intake

To Do:

- ☐
- ☐
- ☐
- ☐
- ☐

Daily Goals:

Date:

Work Out

Exercise	Duration	Intensity

Current Weight ______________________

Met Goals Today?   Yes   No
                      O   O

Notes

____

____

____

____

____

____

____

____

____

	Calories	Carbs	Fat	Protein
Breakfast:				
Lunch:				
Dinner:				
Snack:				
Daily Total:				

Water Intake

To Do:

- ☐
- ☐
- ☐
- ☐
- ☐

Daily Goals:

____

____

____

____

Date:

Work Out

Exercise	Duration	Intensity

Current Weight ________________

Met Goals Today?   Yes   No
                      O   O

Notes

____
____
____
____
____
____
____
____
____
____

	Calories	Carbs	Fat	Protein
Breakfast:				
Lunch:				
Dinner:				
Snack:				
Daily Total:				

Water Intake

To Do:

☐
☐
☐
☐
☐

Daily Goals:

____

____

____

____

Date:

Work Out

Exercise	Duration	Intensity

Current Weight _______________

Met Goals Today?   Yes   No
                     O   O

Notes

____

____

____

____

____

____

____

____

____

	Calories	Carbs	Fat	Protein
Breakfast:				
Lunch:				
Dinner:				
Snack:				
Daily Total:				

Water Intake

To Do:

- ☐
- ☐
- ☐
- ☐
- ☐

Daily Goals:

Date:

Work Out

Exercise	Duration	Intensity

Current Weight _______________

Met Goals Today?   Yes   No
                      O   O

Notes

____

____

____

____

____

____

____

____

____

____

	Calories	Carbs	Fat	Protein
Breakfast:				
Lunch:				
Dinner:				
Snack:				
Daily Total:				

Water Intake

To Do:

- ☐
- ☐
- ☐
- ☐
- ☐

Daily Goals:

____

____

____

____

Date:

Work Out

Exercise	Duration	Intensity

Current Weight _______________

Met Goals Today?   Yes ⭘   No ⭘

Notes

____

____

____

____

____

____

____

____

____

	Calories	Carbs	Fat	Protein
Breakfast:				
Lunch:				
Dinner:				
Snack:				
Daily Total:				

Water Intake

To Do:

- ☐
- ☐
- ☐
- ☐
- ☐

Daily Goals:

Date:

Work Out

Exercise	Duration	Intensity

Current Weight _______________

Met Goals Today?   Yes ⬜   No ⬜

Notes

____

____

____

____

____

____

____

____

____

____

	Calories	Carbs	Fat	Protein
Breakfast:				
Lunch:				
Dinner:				
Snack:				
Daily Total:				

Water Intake

To Do:

- ☐
- ☐
- ☐
- ☐
- ☐

Daily Goals:

Date:

Work Out

Exercise	Duration	Intensity

Current Weight _______________

Met Goals Today?   Yes ◯   No ◯

Notes

____

____

____

____

____

____

____

____

____

	Calories	Carbs	Fat	Protein
Breakfast:				
Lunch:				
Dinner:				
Snack:				
Daily Total:				

Water Intake

To Do:

- ☐
- ☐
- ☐
- ☐
- ☐

Daily Goals:

Work Out

Exercise	Duration	Intensity

Current Weight _______________

Met Goals Today?　　Yes　　No
　　　　　　　　　　　☐　　☐

Notes

____

____

____

____

____

____

____

____

____

	Calories	Carbs	Fat	Protein
Breakfast:				
Lunch:				
Dinner:				
Snack:				
Daily Total:				

Water Intake

To Do:

- ☐
- ☐
- ☐
- ☐
- ☐

Daily Goals:

____

____

____

____

Date:

Work Out

Exercise	Duration	Intensity

Current Weight _______________

Met Goals Today?   Yes ○   No ○

Notes

____

____

____

____

____

____

____

____

____

____

	Calories	Carbs	Fat	Protein
Breakfast:				
Lunch:				
Dinner:				
Snack:				
Daily Total:				

Water Intake

To Do:

☐
☐
☐
☐
☐

Daily Goals:

____

____

____

____

Date:

Work Out

Exercise	Duration	Intensity

Current Weight ______________

Met Goals Today?   Yes ☐   No ☐

Notes

____
____
____
____
____
____
____
____
____

	Calories	Carbs	Fat	Protein
Breakfast:				
Lunch:				
Dinner:				
Snack:				
Daily Total:				

Water Intake

To Do:

- ☐
- ☐
- ☐
- ☐
- ☐

Daily Goals:

Date:

Work Out

Exercise	Duration	Intensity

Current Weight ___________________

Met Goals Today?   Yes   No
                      O   O

Notes

____

____

____

____

____

____

____

____

____

	Calories	Carbs	Fat	Protein
Breakfast:				
Lunch:				
Dinner:				
Snack:				
Daily Total:				

Water Intake

To Do:

- ☐
- ☐
- ☐
- ☐
- ☐

Daily Goals:

____

____

____

____

Date:

Work Out

Exercise	Duration	Intensity

Current Weight _______________

Met Goals Today?   Yes ☐   No ☐

Notes

____
____
____
____
____
____
____
____
____

	Calories	Carbs	Fat	Protein
Breakfast:				
Lunch:				
Dinner:				
Snack:				
Daily Total:				

Water Intake

To Do:

☐
☐
☐
☐
☐

Daily Goals:

____

____

____

____

Work Out

Exercise	Duration	Intensity

Current Weight ________________

Met Goals Today?   Yes ○   No ○

Notes

____

____

____

____

____

____

____

____

____

	Calories	Carbs	Fat	Protein
Breakfast:				
Lunch:				
Dinner:				
Snack:				
Daily Total:				

Water Intake

To Do:

- ☐
- ☐
- ☐
- ☐
- ☐

Daily Goals:

____

____

____

____

Date:

Work Out

Exercise	Duration	Intensity

Current Weight ______________________

Met Goals Today?   Yes ◯   No ◯

Notes

____

____

____

____

____

____

____

____

____

	Calories	Carbs	Fat	Protein
Breakfast:				
Lunch:				
Dinner:				
Snack:				
Daily Total:				

Water Intake

To Do:

☐
☐
☐
☐
☐

Daily Goals:

____

____

____

____

Date:

Work Out

Exercise	Duration	Intensity

Current Weight ___________________

Met Goals Today?   Yes   No
                      O   O

Notes

____

____

____

____

____

____

____

____

____

	Calories	Carbs	Fat	Protein
Breakfast:				
Lunch:				
Dinner:				
Snack:				
Daily Total:				

Water Intake

To Do:

- ☐
- ☐
- ☐
- ☐
- ☐

Daily Goals:

____

____

____

____

Date:

Work Out

Exercise	Duration	Intensity

Current Weight ________________

Met Goals Today?   Yes   No
                      ⃝   ⃝

Notes

____

____

____

____

____

____

____

____

____

	Calories	Carbs	Fat	Protein
Breakfast:				
Lunch:				
Dinner:				
Snack:				
Daily Total:				

Water Intake

To Do:

- [ ]
- [ ]
- [ ]
- [ ]
- [ ]

Daily Goals:

Date:

Work Out

Exercise	Duration	Intensity

Current Weight ___________________

Met Goals Today?   Yes ⬭   No ⬭

Notes

____
____
____
____
____
____
____
____
____
____

	Calories	Carbs	Fat	Protein
Breakfast:				
Lunch:				
Dinner:				
Snack:				
Daily Total:				

Water Intake

To Do:

☐
☐
☐
☐
☐

Daily Goals:

____

____

____

____

Date:

Work Out

Exercise	Duration	Intensity

Current Weight _______________

Met Goals Today?   Yes   No
                     O   O

Notes

____

____

____

____

____

____

____

____

____

____

	Calories	Carbs	Fat	Protein
Breakfast:				
Lunch:				
Dinner:				
Snack:				
Daily Total:				

Water Intake

To Do:

- ☐
- ☐
- ☐
- ☐
- ☐

Daily Goals:

____

____

____

____

Date:

Work Out

Exercise	Duration	Intensity

Current Weight _______________

Met Goals Today?   Yes   No
                      ◯   ◯

Notes

____
____
____
____
____
____
____
____
____

	Calories	Carbs	Fat	Protein
Breakfast:				
Lunch:				
Dinner:				
Snack:				
Daily Total:				

Water Intake

To Do:

- [ ]
- [ ]
- [ ]
- [ ]
- [ ]

Daily Goals:

Date:

Work Out

Exercise	Duration	Intensity

Current Weight _______________

Met Goals Today?   Yes ☐   No ☐

Notes

____

____

____

____

____

____

____

____

____

	Calories	Carbs	Fat	Protein
Breakfast:				
Lunch:				
Dinner:				
Snack:				
Daily Total:				

Water Intake

To Do:

- ☐
- ☐
- ☐
- ☐
- ☐

Daily Goals:

Date:

Work Out

Exercise	Duration	Intensity

Current Weight ________________

Met Goals Today?   Yes ⭘   No ⭘

Notes

____
____
____
____
____
____
____
____
____

	Calories	Carbs	Fat	Protein
Breakfast:				
Lunch:				
Dinner:				
Snack:				
Daily Total:				

Water Intake

To Do:

- ☐
- ☐
- ☐
- ☐
- ☐

Daily Goals:

Date:

Work Out

Exercise	Duration	Intensity

Current Weight ________________

Met Goals Today?   Yes ⬜   No ⬜

Notes

____

____

____

____

____

____

____

____

____

	Calories	Carbs	Fat	Protein
Breakfast:				
Lunch:				
Dinner:				
Snack:				
Daily Total:				

Water Intake

To Do:

- ☐
- ☐
- ☐
- ☐
- ☐

Daily Goals:

____

____

____

____

Date:

Work Out

Exercise	Duration	Intensity

Current Weight ___________________

Met Goals Today?   Yes ⭘   No ⭘

Notes

____

____

____

____

____

____

____

____

____

____

	Calories	Carbs	Fat	Protein
Breakfast:				
Lunch:				
Dinner:				
Snack:				
Daily Total:				

Water Intake

To Do:

- ☐
- ☐
- ☐
- ☐
- ☐

Daily Goals:

____

____

____

____

Date:

Work Out

Exercise	Duration	Intensity

Current Weight _______________

Met Goals Today?   Yes   No
                      ☐   ☐

Notes

____
____
____
____
____
____
____
____
____

	Calories	Carbs	Fat	Protein
Breakfast:				
Lunch:				
Dinner:				
Snack:				
Daily Total:				

Water Intake

To Do:

- ☐
- ☐
- ☐
- ☐
- ☐

Daily Goals:

____

____

____

____

Date:

Work Out

Exercise	Duration	Intensity

Current Weight _______________

Met Goals Today?   Yes ⬭   No ⬭

Notes

____

____

____

____

____

____

____

____

____

	Calories	Carbs	Fat	Protein
Breakfast:				
Lunch:				
Dinner:				
Snack:				
Daily Total:				

Water Intake

To Do:

- ☐
- ☐
- ☐
- ☐
- ☐

Daily Goals:

____

____

____

____

Date:

Work Out

Exercise	Duration	Intensity

Current Weight ___________

Met Goals Today?   Yes ⭘   No ⭘

Notes

____
____
____
____
____
____
____
____
____

	Calories	Carbs	Fat	Protein
Breakfast:				
Lunch:				
Dinner:				
Snack:				
Daily Total:				

Water Intake

To Do:

- ☐
- ☐
- ☐
- ☐
- ☐

Daily Goals:

Date:

Work Out

Exercise	Duration	Intensity

Current Weight ________________

Met Goals Today?   Yes ☐   No ☐

Notes

____
____
____
____
____
____
____
____
____

	Calories	Carbs	Fat	Protein
Breakfast:				
Lunch:				
Dinner:				
Snack:				
Daily Total:				

Water Intake

To Do:

- [ ]
- [ ]
- [ ]
- [ ]
- [ ]

Daily Goals:

____

____

____

____

Date:

Work Out

Exercise	Duration	Intensity

Current Weight _______________

Met Goals Today?   Yes   No
                      ☐   ☐

Notes

____

____

____

____

____

____

____

____

____

	Calories	Carbs	Fat	Protein
Breakfast:				
Lunch:				
Dinner:				
Snack:				
Daily Total:				

Water Intake

To Do:

- ☐
- ☐
- ☐
- ☐
- ☐

Daily Goals:

____

____

____

____

Date:

Work Out

Exercise	Duration	Intensity

Current Weight ___________________

Met Goals Today?   Yes O   No O

Notes

____

____

____

____

____

____

____

____

____

	Calories	Carbs	Fat	Protein
Breakfast:				
Lunch:				
Dinner:				
Snack:				
Daily Total:				

Water Intake

To Do:

- ☐
- ☐
- ☐
- ☐
- ☐

Daily Goals:

Date:

Work Out

Exercise	Duration	Intensity

Current Weight _______________

Met Goals Today?   Yes ☐   No ☐

Notes

____

____

____

____

____

____

____

____

____

	Calories	Carbs	Fat	Protein
Breakfast:				
Lunch:				
Dinner:				
Snack:				
Daily Total:				

Water Intake

To Do:

- ☐
- ☐
- ☐
- ☐
- ☐

Daily Goals:

____

____

____

____

Date:

Work Out

Exercise	Duration	Intensity

Current Weight _______________

Met Goals Today?   Yes O   No O

Notes

____

____

____

____

____

____

____

____

____

	Calories	Carbs	Fat	Protein
Breakfast:				
Lunch:				
Dinner:				
Snack:				
Daily Total:				

Water Intake

To Do:

☐
☐
☐
☐
☐

Daily Goals:

____

____

____

____

Date:

Work Out

Exercise	Duration	Intensity

Current Weight ___________________

Met Goals Today?   Yes ◻   No ◻

Notes

____

____

____

____

____

____

____

____

	Calories	Carbs	Fat	Protein
Breakfast:				
Lunch:				
Dinner:				
Snack:				
Daily Total:				

Water Intake

To Do:

- ☐
- ☐
- ☐
- ☐
- ☐

Daily Goals:

Date:

Work Out

Exercise	Duration	Intensity

Current Weight _______________

Met Goals Today?   Yes   No
                     O   O

Notes

____

____

____

____

____

____

____

____

____

	Calories	Carbs	Fat	Protein
Breakfast:				
Lunch:				
Dinner:				
Snack:				
Daily Total:				

Water Intake

To Do:

- ☐
- ☐
- ☐
- ☐
- ☐

Daily Goals:

____

____

____

____

Date:

Work Out

Exercise	Duration	Intensity

Current Weight ________________

Met Goals Today?   Yes No
                     O   O

Notes

____
____
____
____
____
____
____
____
____

	Calories	Carbs	Fat	Protein
Breakfast:				
Lunch:				
Dinner:				
Snack:				
Daily Total:				

Water Intake

To Do:

- ☐
- ☐
- ☐
- ☐
- ☐

Daily Goals:

____

____

____

____

Date:

Work Out

Exercise	Duration	Intensity

Current Weight _______________

Met Goals Today?   Yes No
                     O   O

Notes

____

____

____

____

____

____

____

____

____

____

	Calories	Carbs	Fat	Protein
Breakfast:				
Lunch:				
Dinner:				
Snack:				
Daily Total:				

Water Intake

To Do:

- ☐
- ☐
- ☐
- ☐
- ☐

Daily Goals:

____

____

____

____

Date:

Work Out

Exercise	Duration	Intensity

Current Weight ___________________

Met Goals Today?   Yes ⬭   No ⬭

Notes

____

____

____

____

____

____

____

____

____

	Calories	Carbs	Fat	Protein
Breakfast:				
Lunch:				
Dinner:				
Snack:				
Daily Total:				

Water Intake

To Do:

- ☐
- ☐
- ☐
- ☐
- ☐

Daily Goals:

____

____

____

____

Date:

Work Out

Exercise	Duration	Intensity

Current Weight _______________

Met Goals Today?   Yes   No
                      O   O

Notes

	Calories	Carbs	Fat	Protein
Breakfast:				
Lunch:				
Dinner:				
Snack:				
Daily Total:				

Water Intake

To Do:

- ☐
- ☐
- ☐
- ☐
- ☐

Daily Goals:

Date:

Work Out

Exercise	Duration	Intensity

Current Weight _______________

Met Goals Today?   Yes   No
                     ⬜   ⬜

Notes

____

____

____

____

____

____

____

____

	Calories	Carbs	Fat	Protein
Breakfast:				
Lunch:				
Dinner:				
Snack:				
Daily Total:				

Water Intake

To Do:

☐
☐
☐
☐
☐

Daily Goals:

Date:

Work Out

Exercise	Duration	Intensity

Current Weight _______________

Met Goals Today?   Yes ⬜   No ⬜

Notes

____

____

____

____

____

____

____

____

____

	Calories	Carbs	Fat	Protein
Breakfast:				
Lunch:				
Dinner:				
Snack:				
Daily Total:				

Water Intake

To Do:

☐
☐
☐
☐
☐

Daily Goals:

Date:

Work Out

Exercise	Duration	Intensity

Current Weight _______________

Met Goals Today?   Yes   No
                      O   O

Notes

____

____

____

____

____

____

____

____

____

	Calories	Carbs	Fat	Protein
Breakfast:				
Lunch:				
Dinner:				
Snack:				
Daily Total:				

Water Intake

To Do:

- ☐
- ☐
- ☐
- ☐
- ☐

Daily Goals:

____

____

____

____

Date:

Work Out

Exercise	Duration	Intensity

Current Weight _________________

Met Goals Today? Yes ◯ No ◯

Notes

____

____

____

____

____

____

____

____

____

	Calories	Carbs	Fat	Protein
Breakfast:				
Lunch:				
Dinner:				
Snack:				
Daily Total:				

Water Intake

To Do:

- ☐
- ☐
- ☐
- ☐
- ☐

Daily Goals:

Date:

Work Out

Exercise	Duration	Intensity

Current Weight ______________

Met Goals Today?   Yes ○   No ○

Notes

____
____
____
____
____
____
____
____
____

	Calories	Carbs	Fat	Protein
Breakfast:				
Lunch:				
Dinner:				
Snack:				
Daily Total:				

Water Intake

To Do:

- [ ]
- [ ]
- [ ]
- [ ]
- [ ]

Daily Goals:

____

____

____

____

Date:

Work Out

Exercise	Duration	Intensity

Current Weight _______________

Met Goals Today?   Yes ◯   No ◯

Notes

____
____
____
____
____
____
____
____
____

	Calories	Carbs	Fat	Protein
Breakfast:				
Lunch:				
Dinner:				
Snack:				
Daily Total:				

Water Intake

To Do:

- ☐
- ☐
- ☐
- ☐
- ☐

Daily Goals:

Work Out

Exercise	Duration	Intensity

Current Weight _______________

Met Goals Today?   Yes   No
                      ☐   ☐

Notes

____

____

____

____

____

____

____

____

____

	Calories	Carbs	Fat	Protein
Breakfast:				
Lunch:				
Dinner:				
Snack:				
Daily Total:				

Water Intake

To Do:

- ☐
- ☐
- ☐
- ☐
- ☐

Daily Goals:

Date:

Work Out

Exercise	Duration	Intensity

Current Weight _______________

Met Goals Today?   Yes   No
                      ☐   ☐

Notes

____

____

____

____

____

____

____

____

____

	Calories	Carbs	Fat	Protein
Breakfast:				
Lunch:				
Dinner:				
Snack:				
Daily Total:				

Water Intake

To Do:

- ☐
- ☐
- ☐
- ☐
- ☐

Daily Goals:

Date:

Work Out

Exercise	Duration	Intensity

Current Weight _______________

Met Goals Today?   Yes ⬜   No ⬜

Notes

____

____

____

____

____

____

____

____

____

	Calories	Carbs	Fat	Protein
Breakfast:				
Lunch:				
Dinner:				
Snack:				
Daily Total:				

Water Intake

To Do:

- ☐
- ☐
- ☐
- ☐
- ☐

Daily Goals:

Date:

Work Out

Exercise	Duration	Intensity

Current Weight ______________

Met Goals Today?   Yes ◯   No ◯

Notes

____

____

____

____

____

____

____

____

	Calories	Carbs	Fat	Protein
Breakfast:				
Lunch:				
Dinner:				
Snack:				
Daily Total:				

Water Intake

To Do:

- ☐
- ☐
- ☐
- ☐
- ☐

Daily Goals:

____

____

____

____

Date:

Work Out

Exercise	Duration	Intensity

Current Weight ___________________

Met Goals Today?   Yes ◯   No ◯

Notes

____

____

____

____

____

____

____

____

____

	Calories	Carbs	Fat	Protein
Breakfast:				
Lunch:				
Dinner:				
Snack:				
Daily Total:				

Water Intake

To Do:

- ☐
- ☐
- ☐
- ☐
- ☐

Daily Goals:

Date:

Work Out

Exercise	Duration	Intensity

Current Weight ______________________

Met Goals Today?   Yes   No
                     O   O

Notes

____
____
____
____
____
____
____
____
____
____

	Calories	Carbs	Fat	Protein
Breakfast:				
Lunch:				
Dinner:				
Snack:				
Daily Total:				

Water Intake

To Do:

- ☐
- ☐
- ☐
- ☐
- ☐

Daily Goals:

____

____

____

____

Date:

Work Out

Exercise	Duration	Intensity

Current Weight _______________

Met Goals Today?   Yes   No
                      ⬜   ⬜

Notes

____

____

____

____

____

____

____

____

____

	Calories	Carbs	Fat	Protein
Breakfast:				
Lunch:				
Dinner:				
Snack:				
Daily Total:				

Water Intake

To Do:

- ☐
- ☐
- ☐
- ☐
- ☐

Daily Goals:

____

____

____

____

Date:

Work Out

Exercise	Duration	Intensity

Current Weight _______________

Met Goals Today?   Yes   No
                      ○   ○

Notes

____
____
____
____
____
____
____
____
____

	Calories	Carbs	Fat	Protein
Breakfast:				
Lunch:				
Dinner:				
Snack:				
Daily Total:				

Water Intake

To Do:

☐
☐
☐
☐
☐

Daily Goals:

Date:

Work Out

Exercise	Duration	Intensity

Current Weight _______________

Met Goals Today?   Yes ☐   No ☐

Notes

____
____
____
____
____
____
____
____
____

	Calories	Carbs	Fat	Protein
Breakfast:				
Lunch:				
Dinner:				
Snack:				
Daily Total:				

Water Intake

To Do:

- ☐
- ☐
- ☐
- ☐
- ☐

Daily Goals:

____

____

____

____

Date:

Work Out

Exercise	Duration	Intensity

Current Weight _______________

Met Goals Today?   Yes   No
                      O   O

Notes

____

____

____

____

____

____

____

____

____

	Calories	Carbs	Fat	Protein
Breakfast:				
Lunch:				
Dinner:				
Snack:				
Daily Total:				

Water Intake

To Do:

☐
☐
☐
☐
☐

Daily Goals:

____

____

____

____

Date:

Work Out

Exercise	Duration	Intensity

Current Weight _______________

Met Goals Today?   Yes ☐   No ☐

Notes

____

____

____

____

____

____

____

____

____

	Calories	Carbs	Fat	Protein
Breakfast:				
Lunch:				
Dinner:				
Snack:				
Daily Total:				

Water Intake

To Do:

- ☐
- ☐
- ☐
- ☐
- ☐

Daily Goals:

Date:

Work Out

Exercise	Duration	Intensity

Current Weight ________________

Met Goals Today?   Yes ☐   No ☐

Notes

____
____
____
____
____
____
____
____
____

	Calories	Carbs	Fat	Protein
Breakfast:				
Lunch:				
Dinner:				
Snack:				
Daily Total:				

Water Intake

To Do:

☐
☐
☐
☐
☐

Daily Goals:

Date:

Work Out

Exercise	Duration	Intensity

Current Weight ___________________

Met Goals Today?   Yes   No
                       O   O

Notes

____

____

____

____

____

____

____

____

	Calories	Carbs	Fat	Protein
Breakfast:				
Lunch:				
Dinner:				
Snack:				
Daily Total:				

Water Intake

To Do:

- ☐
- ☐
- ☐
- ☐
- ☐

Daily Goals:

Date:

Work Out

Exercise	Duration	Intensity

Current Weight ___________________

Met Goals Today?   Yes O   No O

Notes

____

____

____

____

____

____

____

____

____

	Calories	Carbs	Fat	Protein
Breakfast:				
Lunch:				
Dinner:				
Snack:				
Daily Total:				

Water Intake

To Do:

- ☐
- ☐
- ☐
- ☐
- ☐

Daily Goals:

Date:

Work Out

Exercise	Duration	Intensity

Current Weight __________________

Met Goals Today?   Yes   No
                      ☐   ☐

Notes

____

____

____

____

____

____

____

____

____

	Calories	Carbs	Fat	Protein
Breakfast:				
Lunch:				
Dinner:				
Snack:				
Daily Total:				

Water Intake

To Do:

- ☐
- ☐
- ☐
- ☐
- ☐

Daily Goals:

____

____

____

____

Date:

Work Out

Exercise	Duration	Intensity

Current Weight ________________

Met Goals Today?   Yes   No
                     O   O

Notes

____
____
____
____
____
____
____
____
____
____

	Calories	Carbs	Fat	Protein
Breakfast:				
Lunch:				
Dinner:				
Snack:				
Daily Total:				

Water Intake

To Do:

- ☐
- ☐
- ☐
- ☐
- ☐

Daily Goals:

____

____

____

____

Date:

Work Out

Exercise	Duration	Intensity

Current Weight _______________

Met Goals Today?   Yes   No
                     ☐   ☐

Notes

____
____
____
____
____
____
____
____
____

	Calories	Carbs	Fat	Protein
Breakfast:				
Lunch:				
Dinner:				
Snack:				
Daily Total:				

Water Intake

To Do:

☐
☐
☐
☐
☐

Daily Goals:

____

____

____

____

Date:

Work Out

Exercise	Duration	Intensity

Current Weight _______________

Met Goals Today?   Yes O   No O

Notes

	Calories	Carbs	Fat	Protein
Breakfast:				
Lunch:				
Dinner:				
Snack:				
Daily Total:				

Water Intake

To Do:

- [ ]
- [ ]
- [ ]
- [ ]
- [ ]

Daily Goals:

____

____

____

____

Date:

Work Out

Exercise	Duration	Intensity

Current Weight _______________

Met Goals Today?   Yes ◯   No ◯

Notes

____

____

____

____

____

____

____

____

____

	Calories	Carbs	Fat	Protein
Breakfast:				
Lunch:				
Dinner:				
Snack:				
Daily Total:				

Water Intake

To Do:

☐
☐
☐
☐
☐

Daily Goals:

____

____

____

____

Date:

Work Out

Exercise	Duration	Intensity

Current Weight ______________

Met Goals Today?   Yes   No
                      O   O

Notes

____

____

____

____

____

____

____

____

____

	Calories	Carbs	Fat	Protein
Breakfast:				
Lunch:				
Dinner:				
Snack:				
Daily Total:				

Water Intake

To Do:

- [ ]
- [ ]
- [ ]
- [ ]
- [ ]

Daily Goals:

Date:

Work Out

Exercise	Duration	Intensity

Current Weight _______________

Met Goals Today?   Yes   No
                     O   O

Notes

____

____

____

____

____

____

____

____

____

	Calories	Carbs	Fat	Protein
Breakfast:				
Lunch:				
Dinner:				
Snack:				
Daily Total:				

Water Intake

To Do:

- ☐
- ☐
- ☐
- ☐
- ☐

Daily Goals:

Date:

Work Out

Exercise	Duration	Intensity

Current Weight _______________

Met Goals Today?   Yes ◯   No ◯

Notes

____

____

____

____

____

____

____

____

____

	Calories	Carbs	Fat	Protein
Breakfast:				
Lunch:				
Dinner:				
Snack:				
Daily Total:				

Water Intake

To Do:

☐
☐
☐
☐
☐

Daily Goals:

____

____

____

____

Date:

Work Out

Exercise	Duration	Intensity

Current Weight _______________

Met Goals Today?   Yes   No
                      ◯   ◯

Notes

____

____

____

____

____

____

____

____

____

____

	Calories	Carbs	Fat	Protein
Breakfast:				
Lunch:				
Dinner:				
Snack:				
Daily Total:				

Water Intake

To Do:

- ☐
- ☐
- ☐
- ☐
- ☐

Daily Goals:

Date:

Work Out

Exercise	Duration	Intensity

Current Weight ______________

Met Goals Today?   Yes O   No O

Notes

____
____
____
____
____
____
____
____
____

	Calories	Carbs	Fat	Protein
Breakfast:				
Lunch:				
Dinner:				
Snack:				
Daily Total:				

Water Intake

To Do:

- ☐
- ☐
- ☐
- ☐
- ☐

Daily Goals:

____

____

____

____

Date:

Work Out

Exercise	Duration	Intensity

Current Weight _______________

Met Goals Today?   Yes ☐   No ☐

Notes
____
____
____
____
____
____
____
____
____

	Calories	Carbs	Fat	Protein
Breakfast:				
Lunch:				
Dinner:				
Snack:				
Daily Total:				

Water Intake

To Do:

☐
☐
☐
☐
☐

Daily Goals:

Date:

Work Out

Exercise	Duration	Intensity

Current Weight ______________________

Met Goals Today?   Yes   No
                     ○   ○

Notes

____

____

____

____

____

____

____

____

____

	Calories	Carbs	Fat	Protein
Breakfast:				
Lunch:				
Dinner:				
Snack:				
Daily Total:				

Water Intake

To Do:

- ☐
- ☐
- ☐
- ☐
- ☐

Daily Goals:

____

____

____

____

Date:

Work Out

Exercise	Duration	Intensity

Current Weight ______________________

Met Goals Today?   Yes   No
                     ◯   ◯

Notes

____

____

____

____

____

____

____

____

____

	Calories	Carbs	Fat	Protein
Breakfast:				
Lunch:				
Dinner:				
Snack:				
Daily Total:				

Water Intake

To Do:

- ☐
- ☐
- ☐
- ☐
- ☐

Daily Goals:

____

____

____

____

Date:

Work Out

Exercise	Duration	Intensity

Current Weight _______________

Met Goals Today?   Yes   No
                     O   O

Notes

____
____
____
____
____
____
____
____
____

	Calories	Carbs	Fat	Protein
Breakfast:				
Lunch:				
Dinner:				
Snack:				
Daily Total:				

Water Intake

To Do:

- ☐
- ☐
- ☐
- ☐
- ☐

Daily Goals:

____

____

____

____

Date:

Work Out

Exercise	Duration	Intensity

Current Weight   _______________

Met Goals Today?   Yes   No
                      ☐   ☐

Notes

____

____

____

____

____

____

____

____

	Calories	Carbs	Fat	Protein
Breakfast:				
Lunch:				
Dinner:				
Snack:				
Daily Total:				

Water Intake

To Do:

- [ ]
- [ ]
- [ ]
- [ ]
- [ ]

Daily Goals:

____

____

____

____

Date:

Work Out

Exercise	Duration	Intensity

Current Weight _______________

Met Goals Today?   Yes   No
                     O   O

Notes

____
____
____
____
____
____
____
____
____
____

	Calories	Carbs	Fat	Protein
Breakfast:				
Lunch:				
Dinner:				
Snack:				
Daily Total:				

Water Intake

To Do:

- ☐
- ☐
- ☐
- ☐
- ☐

Daily Goals:

____

____

____

____

Date:

Work Out

Exercise	Duration	Intensity

Current Weight _______________

Met Goals Today?   Yes   No
                      O   O

Notes

____
____
____
____
____
____
____
____
____
____

	Calories	Carbs	Fat	Protein
Breakfast:				
Lunch:				
Dinner:				
Snack:				
Daily Total:				

Water Intake

To Do:

☐
☐
☐
☐
☐

Daily Goals:

____

____

____

____

Date:

Work Out

Exercise	Duration	Intensity

Current Weight _______________

Met Goals Today?   Yes ◯   No ◯

Notes

____
____
____
____
____
____
____
____
____

	Calories	Carbs	Fat	Protein
Breakfast:				
Lunch:				
Dinner:				
Snack:				
Daily Total:				

Water Intake

To Do:

☐
☐
☐
☐
☐

Daily Goals:

____
____
____
____

Date:

Work Out

Exercise	Duration	Intensity

Current Weight ___________

Met Goals Today?   Yes   No
                      ⬡   ⬡

Notes

____

____

____

____

____

____

____

____

____

	Calories	Carbs	Fat	Protein
Breakfast:				
Lunch:				
Dinner:				
Snack:				
Daily Total:				

Water Intake

To Do:

☐
☐
☐
☐
☐

Daily Goals:

____

____

____

____

Date:

Work Out

Exercise	Duration	Intensity

Current Weight ________________

Met Goals Today?   Yes   No
                      ◯   ◯

Notes

____

____

____

____

____

____

____

____

____

	Calories	Carbs	Fat	Protein
Breakfast:				
Lunch:				
Dinner:				
Snack:				
Daily Total:				

Water Intake

To Do:

☐
☐
☐
☐
☐

Daily Goals:

____

____

____

____

Date:

Work Out

Exercise	Duration	Intensity

Current Weight _______________

Met Goals Today?   Yes ⃝   No ⃝

Notes

____

____

____

____

____

____

____

____

____

	Calories	Carbs	Fat	Protein
Breakfast:				
Lunch:				
Dinner:				
Snack:				
Daily Total:				

Water Intake

To Do:

- ☐
- ☐
- ☐
- ☐
- ☐

Daily Goals:

____

____

____

____

Date:

Work Out

Exercise	Duration	Intensity

Current Weight   _________________

Met Goals Today?   Yes ⬜   No ⬜

Notes

____

____

____

____

____

____

____

____

____

	Calories	Carbs	Fat	Protein
Breakfast:				
Lunch:				
Dinner:				
Snack:				
Daily Total:				

Water Intake

To Do:

- ☐
- ☐
- ☐
- ☐
- ☐

Daily Goals:

____

____

____

____

Work Out

Exercise	Duration	Intensity

Current Weight __________

Met Goals Today?   Yes ◯   No ◯

Notes

____

____

____

____

____

____

____

____

____

	Calories	Carbs	Fat	Protein
Breakfast:				
Lunch:				
Dinner:				
Snack:				
Daily Total:				

Water Intake

To Do:

☐
☐
☐
☐
☐

Daily Goals:

Date:

Work Out

Exercise	Duration	Intensity

Current Weight _______________

Met Goals Today?   Yes   No
                      O   O

Notes

____

____

____

____

____

____

____

____

____

	Calories	Carbs	Fat	Protein
Breakfast:				
Lunch:				
Dinner:				
Snack:				
Daily Total:				

Water Intake

To Do:

☐
☐
☐
☐
☐

Daily Goals:

____

____

____

____

Date:

Work Out

Exercise	Duration	Intensity

Current Weight _______________

Met Goals Today?   Yes   No
                       O   O

Notes

____

____

____

____

____

____

____

____

____

	Calories	Carbs	Fat	Protein
Breakfast:				
Lunch:				
Dinner:				
Snack:				
Daily Total:				

Water Intake

To Do:

- ☐
- ☐
- ☐
- ☐
- ☐

Daily Goals:

____

____

____

____

Date:

Work Out

Exercise	Duration	Intensity

Current Weight ___________________

Met Goals Today?   Yes ◯   No ◯

Notes

____

____

____

____

____

____

____

____

____

	Calories	Carbs	Fat	Protein
Breakfast:				
Lunch:				
Dinner:				
Snack:				
Daily Total:				

Water Intake

To Do:

- ☐
- ☐
- ☐
- ☐
- ☐

Daily Goals:

____

____

____

____

Date:

Work Out

Exercise	Duration	Intensity

Current Weight _______________

Met Goals Today?   Yes ☐   No ☐

Notes

____

____

____

____

____

____

____

____

____

	Calories	Carbs	Fat	Protein
Breakfast:				
Lunch:				
Dinner:				
Snack:				
Daily Total:				

Water Intake

To Do:

- ☐
- ☐
- ☐
- ☐
- ☐

Daily Goals:

____

____

____

____

Date:

Work Out

Exercise	Duration	Intensity

Current Weight ___________________

Met Goals Today?   Yes   No
                     O   O

Notes

____

____

____

____

____

____

____

____

____

	Calories	Carbs	Fat	Protein
Breakfast:				
Lunch:				
Dinner:				
Snack:				
Daily Total:				

Water Intake

To Do:

- [ ]
- [ ]
- [ ]
- [ ]
- [ ]

Daily Goals:

Date:

Work Out

Exercise	Duration	Intensity

Current Weight   _______________

Met Goals Today?　　Yes ◯　　No ◯

Notes

____

____

____

____

____

____

____

____

____

	Calories	Carbs	Fat	Protein
Breakfast:				
Lunch:				
Dinner:				
Snack:				
Daily Total:				

Water Intake

To Do:

- ☐
- ☐
- ☐
- ☐
- ☐

Daily Goals:

Date:

Work Out

Exercise	Duration	Intensity

Current Weight ___________________

Met Goals Today?   Yes ◯   No ◯

Notes

____

____

____

____

____

____

____

____

____

____

	Calories	Carbs	Fat	Protein
Breakfast:				
Lunch:				
Dinner:				
Snack:				
Daily Total:				

Water Intake

To Do:

- ☐
- ☐
- ☐
- ☐
- ☐

Daily Goals:

____

____

____

____

Date:

Work Out

Exercise	Duration	Intensity

Current Weight _______________

Met Goals Today?   Yes ◯   No ◯

Notes

____

____

____

____

____

____

____

____

	Calories	Carbs	Fat	Protein
Breakfast:				
Lunch:				
Dinner:				
Snack:				
Daily Total:				

Water Intake

To Do:

- ☐
- ☐
- ☐
- ☐
- ☐

Daily Goals:

____

____

____

____

Date:

Work Out

Exercise	Duration	Intensity

Current Weight _______________

Met Goals Today?   Yes   No
                      O   O

Notes

____
____
____
____
____
____
____
____
____
____

	Calories	Carbs	Fat	Protein
Breakfast:				
Lunch:				
Dinner:				
Snack:				
Daily Total:				

Water Intake

To Do:

- [ ]
- [ ]
- [ ]
- [ ]
- [ ]

Daily Goals:

Date:

Work Out

Exercise	Duration	Intensity

Current Weight _______________

Met Goals Today?   Yes   No
                     ◯   ◯

Notes

	Calories	Carbs	Fat	Protein
Breakfast:				
Lunch:				
Dinner:				
Snack:				
Daily Total:				

Water Intake

To Do:

- ☐
- ☐
- ☐
- ☐
- ☐

Daily Goals:

____

____

____

____

Date:

Work Out

Exercise	Duration	Intensity

Current Weight _______________

Met Goals Today?   Yes   No
                      O   O

Notes

____

____

____

____

____

____

____

____

____

	Calories	Carbs	Fat	Protein
Breakfast:				
Lunch:				
Dinner:				
Snack:				
Daily Total:				

Water Intake

To Do:

- ☐
- ☐
- ☐
- ☐
- ☐

Daily Goals:

____

____

____

____

Date:

Work Out

Exercise	Duration	Intensity

Current Weight _______________

Met Goals Today?   Yes ⬭   No ⬭

Notes

____
____
____
____
____
____
____
____
____

	Calories	Carbs	Fat	Protein
Breakfast:				
Lunch:				
Dinner:				
Snack:				
Daily Total:				

Water Intake

To Do:

- ☐
- ☐
- ☐
- ☐
- ☐

Daily Goals:

Date:

Work Out

Exercise	Duration	Intensity

Current Weight ___________________

Met Goals Today?   Yes ⭕   No ⭕

Notes

____

____

____

____

____

____

____

____

____

	Calories	Carbs	Fat	Protein
Breakfast:				
Lunch:				
Dinner:				
Snack:				
Daily Total:				

Water Intake

To Do:

☐
☐
☐
☐
☐

Daily Goals:

Date:

Work Out

Exercise	Duration	Intensity

Current Weight ___________________

Met Goals Today?   Yes ◯   No ◯

Notes

____

____

____

____

____

____

____

____

____

	Calories	Carbs	Fat	Protein
Breakfast:				
Lunch:				
Dinner:				
Snack:				
Daily Total:				

Water Intake

To Do:

- [ ]
- [ ]
- [ ]
- [ ]
- [ ]

Daily Goals:

____

____

____

____

Date:

Work Out

Exercise	Duration	Intensity

Current Weight _______________

Met Goals Today?   Yes   No
                      O   O

Notes

____

____

____

____

____

____

____

____

____

	Calories	Carbs	Fat	Protein
Breakfast:				
Lunch:				
Dinner:				
Snack:				
Daily Total:				

Water Intake

To Do:

- [ ]
- [ ]
- [ ]
- [ ]
- [ ]

Daily Goals:

____

____

____

____

Date:

Work Out

Exercise	Duration	Intensity

Current Weight ________________

Met Goals Today?   Yes ⭘   No ⭘

Notes

____
____
____
____
____
____
____
____
____
____

	Calories	Carbs	Fat	Protein
Breakfast:				
Lunch:				
Dinner:				
Snack:				
Daily Total:				

Water Intake

To Do:

- ☐
- ☐
- ☐
- ☐
- ☐

Daily Goals:

____

____

____

____

Date:

Work Out

Exercise	Duration	Intensity

Current Weight   _______________

Met Goals Today?   Yes ◯   No ◯

Notes

____

____

____

____

____

____

____

____

____

	Calories	Carbs	Fat	Protein
Breakfast:				
Lunch:				
Dinner:				
Snack:				
Daily Total:				

Water Intake

To Do:

☐
☐
☐
☐
☐

Daily Goals:

____

____

____

____

Date:

Work Out

Exercise	Duration	Intensity

Current Weight ___________________

Met Goals Today?   Yes ◯   No ◯

Notes

____

____

____

____

____

____

____

____

____

____

	Calories	Carbs	Fat	Protein
Breakfast:				
Lunch:				
Dinner:				
Snack:				
Daily Total:				

Water Intake

To Do:

☐
☐
☐
☐
☐

Daily Goals:

____

____

____

____

Work Out

Exercise	Duration	Intensity

Current Weight _______________

Met Goals Today?   Yes   No
                     ○   ○

Notes

____

____

____

____

____

____

____

____

____

	Calories	Carbs	Fat	Protein
Breakfast:				
Lunch:				
Dinner:				
Snack:				
Daily Total:				

Water Intake

To Do:

- [ ]
- [ ]
- [ ]
- [ ]
- [ ]

Daily Goals:

Date:

Work Out

Exercise	Duration	Intensity

Current Weight _______________

Met Goals Today?   Yes ⬚   No ⬚

Notes

____

____

____

____

____

____

____

____

____

	Calories	Carbs	Fat	Protein
Breakfast:				
Lunch:				
Dinner:				
Snack:				
Daily Total:				

Water Intake

To Do:

- ☐
- ☐
- ☐
- ☐
- ☐

Daily Goals:

____

____

____

____

Date:

Work Out

Exercise	Duration	Intensity

Current Weight ________________

Met Goals Today?   Yes ⭕   No ⭕

Notes

____

____

____

____

____

____

____

____

____

	Calories	Carbs	Fat	Protein
Breakfast:				
Lunch:				
Dinner:				
Snack:				
Daily Total:				

Water Intake

To Do:

- ☐
- ☐
- ☐
- ☐
- ☐

Daily Goals:

____

____

____

____

Date:

Work Out

Exercise	Duration	Intensity

Current Weight _______________

Met Goals Today?   Yes ◯   No ◯

Notes

____

____

____

____

____

____

____

____

____

	Calories	Carbs	Fat	Protein
Breakfast:				
Lunch:				
Dinner:				
Snack:				
Daily Total:				

Water Intake

To Do:

☐
☐
☐
☐
☐

Daily Goals:

____

____

____

____

Date:

Work Out

Exercise	Duration	Intensity

Current Weight ___________________

Met Goals Today?   Yes   No
                      O   O

Notes

____

____

____

____

____

____

____

____

____

____

	Calories	Carbs	Fat	Protein
Breakfast:				
Lunch:				
Dinner:				
Snack:				
Daily Total:				

Water Intake

To Do:

- ☐
- ☐
- ☐
- ☐
- ☐

Daily Goals:

____

____

____

____

Date:

Work Out

Exercise	Duration	Intensity

Current Weight _______________

Met Goals Today?   Yes ◯   No ◯

Notes

____

____

____

____

____

____

____

____

____

	Calories	Carbs	Fat	Protein
Breakfast:				
Lunch:				
Dinner:				
Snack:				
Daily Total:				

Water Intake

To Do:

- [ ]
- [ ]
- [ ]
- [ ]
- [ ]

Daily Goals:

____

____

____

____

Work Out

Exercise	Duration	Intensity

Current Weight ___________________

Met Goals Today?   Yes ☐   No ☐

Notes

____

____

____

____

____

____

____

____

____

	Calories	Carbs	Fat	Protein
Breakfast:				
Lunch:				
Dinner:				
Snack:				
Daily Total:				

Water Intake

To Do:

☐
☐
☐
☐
☐

Daily Goals:

Date:

Work Out

Exercise	Duration	Intensity

Current Weight __________________

Met Goals Today?   Yes ⬚   No ⬚

Notes

	Calories	Carbs	Fat	Protein
Breakfast:				
Lunch:				
Dinner:				
Snack:				
Daily Total:				

Water Intake

To Do:

☐
☐
☐
☐
☐

Daily Goals:

____

____

____

____

Date:

Work Out

Exercise	Duration	Intensity

Current Weight ___________

Met Goals Today?   Yes ◯   No ◯

Notes

____
____
____
____
____
____
____
____
____
____

	Calories	Carbs	Fat	Protein
Breakfast:				
Lunch:				
Dinner:				
Snack:				
Daily Total:				

Water Intake

To Do:

- ☐
- ☐
- ☐
- ☐
- ☐

Daily Goals:

Work Out

Exercise	Duration	Intensity

Date:

Current Weight ___________

Met Goals Today?   Yes ☐   No ☐

Notes

____

____

____

____

____

____

____

____

____

	Calories	Carbs	Fat	Protein
Breakfast:				
Lunch:				
Dinner:				
Snack:				
Daily Total:				

Water Intake

To Do:

☐
☐
☐
☐
☐

Daily Goals:

____
____
____
____

Date:

Work Out

Exercise	Duration	Intensity

Current Weight _______________

Met Goals Today?   Yes ◯   No ◯

Notes

____

____

____

____

____

____

____

____

____

____

	Calories	Carbs	Fat	Protein
Breakfast:				
Lunch:				
Dinner:				
Snack:				
Daily Total:				

Water Intake

To Do:

- ☐
- ☐
- ☐
- ☐
- ☐

Daily Goals:

Date:

Work Out

Exercise	Duration	Intensity

Current Weight _______________

Met Goals Today?   Yes ⭕   No ⭕

Notes

____

____

____

____

____

____

____

____

____

	Calories	Carbs	Fat	Protein
Breakfast:				
Lunch:				
Dinner:				
Snack:				
Daily Total:				

Water Intake

To Do:

- ☐
- ☐
- ☐
- ☐
- ☐

Daily Goals:

____

____

____

____

Work Out

Exercise	Duration	Intensity

Current Weight ______________

Met Goals Today?   Yes ⬜   No ⬜

Notes

____
____
____
____
____
____
____
____
____
____

	Calories	Carbs	Fat	Protein
Breakfast:				
Lunch:				
Dinner:				
Snack:				
Daily Total:				

Water Intake

To Do:

- [ ]
- [ ]
- [ ]
- [ ]
- [ ]

Daily Goals:

Date:

Work Out

Exercise	Duration	Intensity

Current Weight _______________

Met Goals Today?   Yes ◯   No ◯

Notes

____

____

____

____

____

____

____

____

____

	Calories	Carbs	Fat	Protein
Breakfast:				
Lunch:				
Dinner:				
Snack:				
Daily Total:				

Water Intake

To Do:

- ☐
- ☐
- ☐
- ☐
- ☐

Daily Goals:

____

____

____

____

Date:

Work Out

Exercise	Duration	Intensity

Current Weight _______________

Met Goals Today?   Yes ⬜   No ⬜

Notes

____

____

____

____

____

____

____

____

____

	Calories	Carbs	Fat	Protein
Breakfast:				
Lunch:				
Dinner:				
Snack:				
Daily Total:				

Water Intake

To Do:

- ☐
- ☐
- ☐
- ☐
- ☐

Daily Goals:

<h1>Date:</h1>

Work Out

Exercise	Duration	Intensity

Current Weight ___________________

Met Goals Today?   Yes ◯   No ◯

Notes

____

____

____

____

____

____

____

____

____

	Calories	Carbs	Fat	Protein
Breakfast:				
Lunch:				
Dinner:				
Snack:				
Daily Total:				

Water Intake

To Do:

- [ ]
- [ ]
- [ ]
- [ ]
- [ ]

Daily Goals:

____

____

____

____

Date:

Work Out

Exercise	Duration	Intensity

Current Weight _______________

Met Goals Today?   Yes ⬜   No ⬜

Notes

____

____

____

____

____

____

____

____

	Calories	Carbs	Fat	Protein
Breakfast:				
Lunch:				
Dinner:				
Snack:				
Daily Total:				

Water Intake

To Do:

- [ ]
- [ ]
- [ ]
- [ ]
- [ ]

Daily Goals:

____

____

____

____

Date:

Work Out

Exercise	Duration	Intensity

Current Weight _______________

Met Goals Today?   Yes ◯   No ◯

Notes

____

____

____

____

____

____

____

____

	Calories	Carbs	Fat	Protein
Breakfast:				
Lunch:				
Dinner:				
Snack:				
Daily Total:				

Water Intake

To Do:

- ☐
- ☐
- ☐
- ☐
- ☐

Daily Goals:

Work Out

Exercise	Duration	Intensity

Current Weight ______________

Met Goals Today?   Yes ◯   No ◯

Notes

____

____

____

____

____

____

____

____

____

	Calories	Carbs	Fat	Protein
Breakfast:				
Lunch:				
Dinner:				
Snack:				
Daily Total:				

Water Intake

To Do:

- [ ]
- [ ]
- [ ]
- [ ]
- [ ]

Daily Goals:

Date:

Work Out

Exercise	Duration	Intensity

Current Weight ________________

Met Goals Today?   Yes ◯   No ◯

Notes

____

____

____

____

____

____

____

____

____

	Calories	Carbs	Fat	Protein
Breakfast:				
Lunch:				
Dinner:				
Snack:				
Daily Total:				

Water Intake

To Do:

- ☐
- ☐
- ☐
- ☐
- ☐

Daily Goals:

Date:

Work Out

Exercise	Duration	Intensity

Current Weight ______________

Met Goals Today?   Yes ☐   No ☐

Notes

____
____
____
____
____
____
____
____
____

	Calories	Carbs	Fat	Protein
Breakfast:				
Lunch:				
Dinner:				
Snack:				
Daily Total:				

Water Intake

To Do:

- ☐
- ☐
- ☐
- ☐
- ☐

Daily Goals:

Date:

Work Out

Exercise	Duration	Intensity

Current Weight _______________

Met Goals Today? Yes ◯ No ◯

Notes

____

____

____

____

____

____

____

____

____

	Calories	Carbs	Fat	Protein
Breakfast:				
Lunch:				
Dinner:				
Snack:				
Daily Total:				

Water Intake

To Do:

- ☐
- ☐
- ☐
- ☐
- ☐

Daily Goals:

Date:

Work Out

Exercise	Duration	Intensity

Current Weight _______________

Met Goals Today? Yes ◯ No ◯

Notes

____

____

____

____

____

____

____

____

____

____

	Calories	Carbs	Fat	Protein
Breakfast:				
Lunch:				
Dinner:				
Snack:				
Daily Total:				

Water Intake

To Do:

- [ ]
- [ ]
- [ ]
- [ ]
- [ ]

Daily Goals:

Date:

Work Out

Exercise	Duration	Intensity

Current Weight ______________

Met Goals Today?   Yes ⃝   No ⃝

Notes

____

____

____

____

____

____

____

____

____

	Calories	Carbs	Fat	Protein
Breakfast:				
Lunch:				
Dinner:				
Snack:				
Daily Total:				

Water Intake

To Do:

- [ ]
- [ ]
- [ ]
- [ ]
- [ ]

Daily Goals:

____

____

____

____

Date:

Work Out

Exercise	Duration	Intensity

Current Weight _______________

Met Goals Today?   Yes ⭕   No ⭕

Notes

____
____
____
____
____
____
____
____
____

	Calories	Carbs	Fat	Protein
Breakfast:				
Lunch:				
Dinner:				
Snack:				
Daily Total:				

Water Intake

To Do:

- ☐
- ☐
- ☐
- ☐
- ☐

Daily Goals:

Date:

Work Out

Exercise	Duration	Intensity

Current Weight ______________________

Met Goals Today?   Yes ⬜   No ⬜

Notes

____

____

____

____

____

____

____

____

____

	Calories	Carbs	Fat	Protein
Breakfast:				
Lunch:				
Dinner:				
Snack:				
Daily Total:				

Water Intake

To Do:

- ☐
- ☐
- ☐
- ☐
- ☐

Daily Goals:

Date:

Work Out

Exercise	Duration	Intensity

Current Weight _______________

Met Goals Today?   Yes ◯   No ◯

Notes

____

____

____

____

____

____

____

____

____

	Calories	Carbs	Fat	Protein
Breakfast:				
Lunch:				
Dinner:				
Snack:				
Daily Total:				

Water Intake

To Do:

- [ ]
- [ ]
- [ ]
- [ ]
- [ ]

Daily Goals:

Date:

Work Out

Exercise	Duration	Intensity

Current Weight _______________

Met Goals Today?   Yes ☐   No ☐

Notes

____

____

____

____

____

____

____

____

____

	Calories	Carbs	Fat	Protein
Breakfast:				
Lunch:				
Dinner:				
Snack:				
Daily Total:				

Water Intake

To Do:

- ☐
- ☐
- ☐
- ☐
- ☐

Daily Goals:

Date: _______

Work Out

Exercise	Duration	Intensity

Current Weight _______________________

Met Goals Today?   Yes ⬜   No ⬜

Notes

____

____

____

____

____

____

____

____

____

____

www.ingramcontent.com/pod-product-compliance
Lightning Source LLC
Chambersburg PA
CBHW081929270726
48658CB00007BA/2414